I0407159

The information in this book is for educational and entertainment purposes only. It is based on my personal experience, my direct and sustained observations, and my interpretation of research.

I am not a doctor or trained medical professional, and I do not have any knowledge of your health history, (physical or mental) and therefore no knowledge of your individual circumstances.

Before you begin this, or any, fitness program, you should consult with your physician. They can evaluate the potential negative impacts of a change in exercise or diet. I can't.

Table of Contents

Welcome to Las Vegas!

We've all seen that sign. You know the one I'm talking about. It's that "Welcome to Las Vegas" sign used in almost every advertisement for Sin City.

That sign speaks of hope. Liberation. Crazy good times that happen in Vegas and . . . stay in Vegas.

But for many this sign also speaks of insecurity.

Wearing a t-shirt over your bathing suit.

Holding your breath to suck in fat while trying to look confident as you talk to your Sin City associates.

Hoping nobody posted pictures on Facebook, or perhaps frantically "untagging" or disapproving the ones taken while you were exhaling.

That's just not fun, which is the whole point of a vacation, right? It's hard to enjoy yourself and sling witty comments when your diaphragm is cramping from sucking in your gut all day.

You never have to feel that way again--if you don't want to.

Whether your next vacation is in seven weeks, seven months, or seven days, I'm going to give you a smart, effective, and completely achievable plan that will have you confidently relaxing by the pool and having carefree fun—which is what you came for.

The programs in this book are designed to focus on well-tested and effective approaches to short- or long-term results. They're based on decades of research, personal and shared trials, and feedback from readers like you.

You'll follow your plan because you'll know **why** it is going to work. And knowing why it works will help you follow it during those times you don't want to.

Most people don't live to be fit. They want to be fit to help make living better. My goal is to get you to your goal, and then let you get on living your life.

I will not leave you hanging, upsell more programs, or try to keep you coming back. (There's a reason that happens a lot in this industry, which I share in a later chapter.)

For now, let's just focus on my 5-step plan to get fit for Vegas:

1. You read this book.
2. You pick a plan and follow it.
3. You give me feedback that lets me know what parts of the book are helpful.
4. You get fit.
5. We leave each other alone.

If you're in, then . . . ante up!

If you liked this Chapter, please:

Click this link: http://fitfor.lv/uWGcDL

or scan the QR Code below:

How to read this book

3 easy ways to help others get fit:

1. Click a link at the end of each chapter
2. Write a review
3. Get a gift

To help me help you and others, I'm going to ask you do something you've probably never done when reading a book before: click a link. Or take a picture. Yes, a picture.

You'll notice there is a link at the end of each chapter. If you like a chapter, I am asking that you click on that link. It'll do two things:

1. It'll let me track automatically if that chapter was helpful to you.
2. It'll take you to the page on amazon.com where you can choose to write a review.

Why am I asking you to do this? The first item helps me track which chapters are the most helpful to readers. I'll watch and note which chapters get clicks, and the ones that don't, and will use that to assist me in fine-tuning future versions of this book. Think of this as an in-book version of the "Like" button you see on Facebook.

The second item tells others what you think.

And by the way, 5-star reviews will help this book stand out among all the other bazillion fitness books on amazon.com, which will in turn help me get more feedback on this program.

So, if you are enjoying this book, even if you don't think it's perfect, please consider a 5-star review. You will help make it better over time due to the increased feedback and your input will help me fine-tune it.

I know writing a review takes time, so after you do, drop me an e-mail (bruce@fitforvegas.com) and show me your review - I'll personally send you a special thank-you gift. I promise.

I mentioned you could take a picture as well. You've now seen the black and white squares at the end of each chapter. These squares are "QR Codes." They're like bar codes. If you have smart phone, you can take a picture of the square, and if you have the right software on the phone, it'll "scan" this code and automatically "click" a link for you. Most smart phones come ready to do this when you point your camera at one of the black squares. But if yours doesn't you can use the link below to install an app that does this. This is one of the popular QR Code readers, and the program at this address will auto-detect the right app for your phone.

http://fitforvegas.com/links/qrreader.html

Clicking links with your phone in this manner is especially helpful if you want to provide feedback, but not navigate away from the page you're currently reading.

If you liked this Chapter, please:

Click this link: http://fitfor.lv/s43MEE

or scan the QR Code below:

Not about me

Every fitness book I've ever read has had a chapter about the author which serves to qualify the author to the reader. It says something like, "Yes, dear reader, I too have been like you. I too wanted to get fit for Vegas. And guess what, I did!" And then it goes into deep detail with case studies, personal anecdotes, and third party attestations into how it works and why they have the secret ingredients to a fitness plan that works when the multitudes of others have failed. When I've read them, I've always had a little voice in the back of my mind that says something like, "I think he likes himself too much. And he thinks he is just a unique little snowflake, doesn't he? Please, sir, just help me get fit. Thank you."

So here's my "About Me" section:

- I used to be out of shape.
- Now I am in shape.
- I got in shape while having a real job and a very busy life.

I'm actually in pretty amazing shape, and it feels great and I'm super-thankful. So I don't mind investing some time in sharing what worked for me, and what worked for others, so you can do it too. I probably won't make much, if any, money in writing this book.

That's okay. If I get feedback that it works, that's enough for me. It's not my primary form of income, and I don't expect it to be.

However, if you do want the personal anecdotes, and more detail into who I am and why I am qualified to write a book like this, I put that at the end of the book. Like all the other authors, I *do* like myself. And *I do* think I'm a unique snowflake. My mom told me so, and I've always believed her. I'm just not so full of myself to make it a big ol' chapter at the start of the book.

If you liked this Chapter, please:

Click this link: http://fitfor.lv/rZKsvi

or scan the QR Code below:

The basics - Society wants you to be fat.

It's simple to get fit. But it's not easy. In fact, it's pretty damn hard. Probably not exactly what you wanted to hear, but it's the truth. That's why there are so many people that are *not* in shape. But here's the deal: once you "get it" then it becomes a hell of a lot easier. But there are so many myths and misconceptions out there, most

> **Common Sense Rule #1**
>
> If getting fit were easy, then you'd know more people that were actually fit.

created by a lot of well-meaning people, that it gets super-hard to focus on what actually works. I've even seen people get fit, experience a lot of success being fit, and slip back into doing what doesn't work and get fat again. This is mostly because what they thought was the secret to getting fit the first time was actually just a happy coincidence rather than doing what permanently works.

To help you focus on what works, let me first explain why getting fit is hard.

It all starts with the fact that society wants you to be fat.

Humans have been around a long time. Anyone that's read up on the "paleo diet" knows that the modern diet is only a few thousand years old at best, and therefore new to our bodies in an evolutionary sense. According to the "paleo diet" that's why we get fat. There is a lot of truth to this theory. But that's not the main reason so many people are overweight in modern society. We're fat because of two things:

- Your body wants to have "just enough" muscle for you to hunt food and defend yourself from enemies.
- Your body wants you to have plenty of fat in case you go a while without finding or hunting food

For most of mankind's existence, food was hard to come by, and living was tough. Getting food and fending off wild animals was a full-time job. And muscle, for all its glamour on modern magazine covers, was a liability for most ancient men. That's because just having muscle increases the calories you burn, and that depletes your food stores. As a result if ancient man ran out of food (like when you diet), muscle was the first thing his body would burn for energy. Fat, on the other hand, doesn't take much fuel to maintain. And his body could live off of that if he couldn't hunt or find food. And to set that ancient man up for success, the foods that had the most chance of making him fat, specifically those that were calorie dense or easy to eat a lot of, were also the ones that tasted the best! This isn't an evil trick by a fat bastard demon. It's smart . . . if you're a caveman. Because fat cavemen, with just enough muscle to run and kill that tiger and haul it to the cave, were the ones that lived on to become old cavemen.

But modern man doesn't really *have* to do a lot of walking or heavy lifting to get food. So we won't build muscle unless we simulate that kind of activity by getting on a treadmill or lifting weights. And our taste buds haven't changed that much in the last few thousand years. The fatty stuff still tastes the best. Modern fats like butter, fried food, processed carbs, sugary sweets--all these foods either have loads of calories in each serving or make us want to eat even more. And it's not just the fast food nation that packs on the calories. Even at gourmet restaurants, the food is usually cooked in high quality oils or covered with buttery sauces to keep you a happy (and fatty) customer.

So you can see we are set up for failure. Our bodies are programmed to get rid of muscle when we diet, and our mental state encourages us to eat the foods that are most likely to make us fat. And in modern society, that kind of food is all around us. That is why I say, "Society wants us to be fat."

This is the main reason why getting fit is so difficult. In order to counter-act this programing, every day, or at least more days than not, you have to set yourself up to:

- Trick your body into thinking it needs more muscle to survive
- Eat less calories than you use each day, which means not eating the food that tastes the best

The good news? You don't have to be perfect. You don't have to be in the gym all day. And you don't have to deny yourself the great-tasting foods. But you do have to do these two things more days than you don't do them if you ever want to truly get fit in time for Vegas.

If you liked this Chapter, please:

Click this link: http://fitfor.lv/uwA5aT

or scan the QR Code below:

Diet - You can't outrun a pizza

Since we're talking about diet in this chapter, I'll start with a pizza. But it's not a real pizza. It's a pizza pie chart. I lovingly call it the "fat kid pie of cold hard truth".

the fat kid pie of cold hard truth

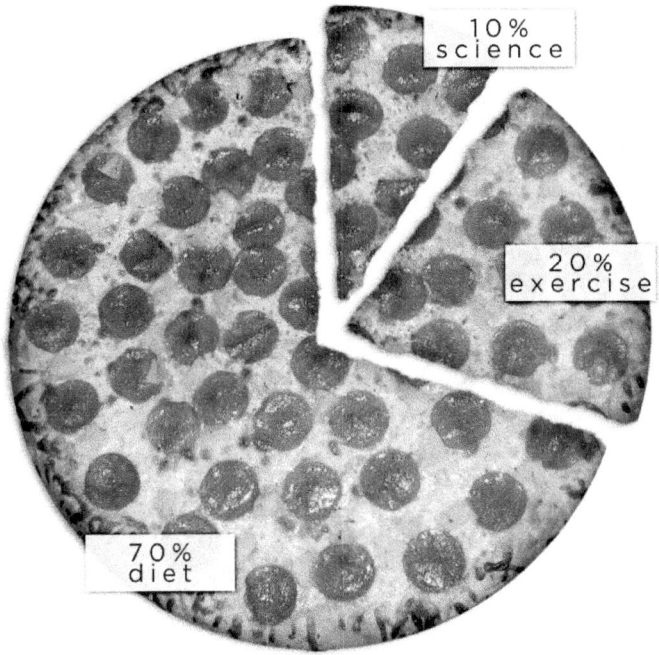

10% science

20% exercise

70% diet

The chart in this chapter shows the three components of fitness, and their relative importance. The first component is diet, and it is the most important component to getting fit, and thus it makes up 70% of the pie. Exercise is 20%. The third component, science, makes up the remaining 10% of the solution. I'll go more into how science can help you get fit in a later chapter. I call this the "fat kid pie of cold hard truth" because many people trying to get fit would like to think that some other parts of the pie, like exercise, or science, can help more than diet. But, unfortunately, that's not the case. And I'll explain why in this chapter.

There are a few really good reasons why diet is 70% of the pie. First of all, you have to control your diet almost all day and all night. You only need to go to the gym a few hours a week. Second, you're tempted to eat junk food almost all day and all night, but you're only tempted to *not* work out during those few hours you're *supposed* to workout. But the third reason, and this is the most important, is that no matter who you are . . . you can't outrun a pizza.

Explanation – You need to understand that you lose weight if you eat fewer calories than you burn. Its simple thermodynamics, which basically means energy doesn't just disappear. It has to go somewhere. When you eat calories, you are taking energy into your body. And it has to go somewhere. It's going into one of two places. Either into "heat," in the form of work you do moving your body around, or into "matter" in the form of fat or muscle. In fact, the whole concept behind a calorie is that it is a measure of energy. And, for 99.99% of the world out there – if you eat about 7,000 fewer calories than you burn a week, you'll lose almost exactly two pounds of solid fat each week. Really. You might lose more depending on your diet, and that's almost always due to the amount of water you're storing within your body. But at 7,000 fewer calories a week, which is about the most you can lose without losing a lot of muscle too, you'll drop 2 pounds of real fat off your body each week, guaranteed. And that can start to really change how you look in a bathing suit. No drugs, supplements, or other science needed.

Now, there is some science and there are some supplements that can make a diet more or less than 70% of the solution, but at most these factors will impact your overall fitness by about 10%. And depending on what you eat, you'll either lose more fat or lose more muscle. But there's no amount of science, or specialty diet, or drug that will have you losing weight if you eat more than you burn. That goes for every single popular diet you have ever heard of. The South Beach diet works because it focuses on low glycemic carbs that kill off the feedback loop that makes you hungry and eat more food, so you take in fewer overall calories. The "slow carb" diet from Tim Ferriss's *Four Hour Body* does much of the same. The Atkins diet works because it cuts out one of the 3 major types of macro nutrients, carbs, and when you do that, you eat fewer calories--about a third less, in fact. And the "paleo diet" works because no matter who you are, you can't sit down and eat a bowl full of apples and stacks of lean meat, and so you also eat fewer calories. Weight Watchers™ works because they monitor 'calories in' vs. 'calories out' through their point system. They all have special optimizations that help make them easier to stick with, but they all, ultimately, help you eat less.

Now, some of the astute readers might ask, "But can't I quickly burn a bunch of calories, and thus lose more fat, faster?" Good question. I know many people who, after they break down and eat some really high-calorie (but wonderfully tasty) food, like a pizza, make themselves feel better by proclaiming, "Well, I'll do an extra mile during my run tomorrow." That's not going to work.

Yes, you can increase how many calories you burn through exercise, or through increasing your activity every day. And this can help accelerate fat loss. That's why exercise makes up 20% of the "fat kid pie". But you cannot out-exercise a bad diet.

I realized this when I ran my first marathon. It was, and remains, a once-in-a-lifetime event. I ran a fairly steady pace for 26.2 miles, and walked only a couple miles due to injury, and in the end finished at a blistering 4 hours and change. I also wore a device that tracks calorie burn with 95% accuracy. I burned a total of 2,642 calories during my marathon. Now, what is the total calorie count if you sit down and eat one large pizza? On average, the answer is 2,700 calories.

How many marathons have you ran? How many pizzas have you eaten? It's a safe bet, even in Vegas, that you've eaten many more pizzas than run marathons.

You can't out-exercise a bad diet. But you can create a diet that sets you up for success. And how aggressive that diet will be depends a lot on how much time you've given yourself to hit your target.

In each of the three weight-loss programs I outline in this book, a diet is designed that focuses on achieving the best results in the time you've given yourself to get fit for Vegas.

If you liked this Chapter, please:

Click this link: http://fitfor.lv/vnu0Bl

or scan the QR Code below:

Exercise – why sweat it?

This is actually a big, scary, complex topic for a lot of people. With workouts with names like Insanity™, P90x™, Zumba ™, CrossFit™, and personal trainers and gyms running multiple classes and hundreds of machines per gym, why wouldn't it be? But you don't need to sweat it because I'm going to break this down into three simple parts. Let me point something out. Take a look around the gym next time you're there. Do the fittest men and women also look the most intelligent? Does it look like they've solved some complex physiological problems? Conversely, think about the smartest people you know. Are they the most fit? There are certainly exceptions to this generalization. Not all fit people are "boneheads", and not all smart people are out of shape. But, regardless of intelligence, the super-fit people are the ones that follow a consistent

> **Common Sense Rule #2**
>
> If exercising was really complicated, only really smart people would be fit.

approach and know what their goal is when they go in the gym. So exercise need not be too complex to be effective.

People who know about working out, do it for three reasons – to lose weight by burning some extra calories each day, to build additional muscle through strength-training, and to increase their cardiovascular (heart) health through cardio.

When you exercise, you're going to gain improved cardiovascular health by doing either of the first two activities with any degree of intensity.

Most people focus on cardio, like running, the elliptical machine, or stair stepper, when they want to "burn calories." But you can also burn nearly that many calories doing strength training. And since strength training focuses on building muscle, this is what people really need to do when they want to get "toned" or "ripped." For this reason, I'll be focusing primarily on exercises that build strength and muscle tone, while burning some extra calories at the same time.

There are some strength training basics that you should learn to help understand the workouts in the book—or those in any fitness magazine, or of any fit people you may know who might explain their own routines to you.

1. "Reps" are a single motion of an exercise.
2. "Sets" are a group of those reps. Most "sets" are 8 to 15 "Reps"
3. "Splits" are how you break up a workout to cover different body parts over the course of a week. A typical "split" is a Monday, Tuesday, Thursday, Friday split – where you focus on Back, Arms, Legs and Chest on each of those days respectively. There are many, many split combinations.

How you combine reps and sets and splits depends on how much time you've given yourself to get fit for Vegas. And in each of my programs, I've picked the best set of exercises, and modifications, to make the most of the time you've given yourself.

A couple important points as you get ready to exercise. First – check with a doctor to make sure you don't have any outstanding health issues. Second - doing the exercise correctly is important, especially so you don't hurt yourself. But doing any exercise at all is better than none, so don't get stressed about perfection. With the knowledge I've just provided, and some simple online resources I've provided in each program, you can strength train effectively and achieve amazing results.

However, if you are a perfectionist, or if you want take a more advanced approach, there are two things I'd recommend. One is getting a personal trainer. They help keep you coming to the gym, and they will help you get the most out of each exercise by checking your form and pushing you harder on each rep. You'll see that I recommend one for the first 7 weeks of the 7 month program. They are a great asset, but you don't need to keep them around for every workout, or for over a year. If you're hanging out with them 4-5 days a week for over a year, then they're a rent-a-friend, not a trainer. And they aren't cheap. Get a real friend and bring them to the gym - they'll thank you for the workouts.

Secondly, if you would rather have the classroom feel, CrossFit™, which exploded onto the fitness scene in the last 5 years, is actually a very well-structured workout plan. CrossFit™ instructors work closely with new and novice members on form and technique, which can help keep you safe, and also break the fear barrier in lifting weights. Each CrossFit™ gym usually builds a community feel and the workouts are structured in a way where you compete with yourself. This clever combination makes it hard to stay away too long, and keeps you wanting to come back. And as I said in the last chapter, since you need to do the two simple steps more days than you don't, this is a great formula for success. If you're brand spanking new to working out, or it's been a while, check with your doc, and I'd highly recommend getting a handful of personal training or at least one intro session to CrossFit™. Not only is it safer, but it also will make you a hell of a lot more comfortable when you work out on your own.

If you liked this Chapter, please:

Click this link: http://fitfor.lv/s3J2yo

or scan the QR Code below:

Tools – The Six Sigma method to getting ripped and toned

Peter Drucker, one of the most well-known thinkers in optimizing business processes, is rumored to have once said, "If you can't measure it, you can't manage it." And this same principle has been used in businesses world-wide to improve complex processes, and keep track of difficult to achieve targets and goals. So, if it works for the Fortune 100 companies, why wouldn't it work for you? Heck, even in Vegas, gamblers adopt this mantra when they count cards to increase their odds for success.

> **Common Sense Rule #3**
>
> Really fit people know about how many calories they eat each day.
>
> (Ask one. They'll tell you.)

Adopting a "measuring" approach to getting fit helps you stay on track, shows progress before you see it in the mirror, and shows what progress you will lose if you backslide. I've been measuring my calorie intake, output, weight, body fat, and body circumference for over four years. And while I don't take measurements all the time or every day, I do this more days than I don't. And if I added up all the time I spend measuring each week, it'd be about 20 minutes total. This has been my Number One Success Factor in getting fit. You could spend a lot more time measuring things than I do. To save you the research and money, below is a short list of tools I've used on my trek to getting fit. I make no money if you buy these. These are just the ones that work the best based on my own personal experience and feedback from trusted friends and fitness pros.

Measure calories burned: almost every day

- BodyMedia FIT (http://fitfor.lv/uQXf6T)– this is an armband that tracks your calorie burn. It's 95% accurate. You've probably seen it on the TV show, The Biggest Loser ™. It requires a subscription to a website, but it's a well-designed site that also helps you log the food you eat.
- If you don't want to pay, you can estimate your calories burned with many online calorie burn estimators, and log it in a free site – fitday.com.
- One thing I wouldn't recommend – heart rate monitors. They guess calorie burn by assuming a lot about why your heart rate is going up. I've seen these be off by 500 calories in a single workout. That's the difference of losing or gaining a pound of fat in a week. Trust fitday.com before you trust these.

Measure calories in: almost every day

- BodyMedia FIT (http://fitfor.lv/uQXf6T)– as I mentioned above, this website and arm band not only measure calories burned, but also helps track calories eaten through an effective food logging application.
- If you don't want to shell out the dough – then you can just log food on fitday.com – a free site.

Check or measure weight: daily or at least weekly.

- Withings WiFi Scale (http://fitfor.lv/vXsGun) – Stand on the scale each day. It uploads your weight to a private website Then one day look back at the trends online. It's just that easy.

- If you don't want to pay for the tech, get any scale. Just use it the same time every day. I recommend early AM right after your first good morning bathroom break.

Body Circumference Measurement: weekly.

Measure what you care most about growing or shrinking. Generally that's arms, waist, and chest. If you want to grow something else, that's a different book. Make sure you measure the same way every time. I do this by flexing the muscle group I'm measuring as hard as I can. I can consistently flex as hard as I can each time I measure. I can't "relax" as consistently, especially because I find myself flexing "just a bit" to cheat my own numbers.

- Myotape (http://fitfor.lv/sXDmGc) – it's a measuring tape that you can use with one hand, so you don't have to be embarrassed by having somebody help you wrap the thing around your large gut or skinny bicep.
- If you don't want to pay for that, use a shoestring. Hold the two measure points. Measure those points with a ruler. But c'mon. Really? Just buy the thingy above. It's probably 10 bucks or so.

Measure Body Fat Percentage: weekly.

This is actually the most important measurement. Because all the above don't tell you the difference between fat and muscle. And believe me, you're going for more muscle than fat. Typically, guys that are "ripped" are under 10% and more often 6% or less. For women that have some abs, they are under 15%. Any lower, and you're going to hurt yourself. A good, accurate, measurement in this area will be a true measure of progress.

- Hydrostatic Body Fat Test (http://fitfor.lv/vlq6ll) – there are many ways to measure body fat. The hydrostatic (dunk-tank) is the gold standard way to test. I thought I'd have to go to some high-tech university to use one of these, but it turns out, for $50 or so you can do this if you follow the schedule on this site.
- BodyMetrix (http://fitfor.lv/vL084r) – this new clever device is a bit pricier, but almost as accurate as the dunk tank. It uses ultrasound to upload fat thickness to your PC. Dead easy to use. And gives you all kinds of ways to measure fat in problem areas. I love mine.
- Skin fold calipers (http://fitfor.lv/sXDmGc) – less accurate, as they depend a lot on somebody pinching you in the same way each time, and you can't do these on your own. If you get a trainer, have them do this each week for you.
- Body fat scales – even my favorite Withings scale sucks in trying to guess body fat percentage. And it varies a lot with how much water you drank in the hours before you stepped on it. So I'd not even recommend using these at all.

Record each of these in a spreadsheet and you can make cool graphs to impress your friends. I've got a sample from a workout push I did the summer of 2011 included in the figure below. It shows how I tracked these measurements, and used the information from the previous chapter to track where I should be compared to where I am.

Date	Cals in	Cals out	Cals Net	Weight	Body Fat	Waist Fat Thickne	Target Weight	Target Body Fat
7/18/2011	1601	3597	1996	182.9	9.30%	6.9	183	12.00%
7/19/2011	1816	3599	1783	177.6	9.10%	7.6	178	11.98%
7/20/2011	1448	3174	1726	175.9	8.10%	5.8	178	9.17%
7/21/2011	4009	3009	-1000	177.6	8.10%	6.6	177	9.00%
7/22/2011	1674	3448	1774	178.7	8.60%	6.8	177	8.83%
7/23/2011	2112	3790	1678	174.9	8.20%	6.7	177	8.66%
7/24/2011	5095	4453	-642	175.7	8.00%	6.2	176	8.49%
7/25/2011	1614	2718	1104	177.5	8.10%	6.2	176	8.32%
7/26/2011	1938	2717	779	174.7	7.70%	5.9	176	8.16%
7/27/2011	2274	3063	789	174.9	7.90%	6.4	176	7.99%
7/28/2011	1932	3450	1518	175.2	7.80%	5.9	175	7.82%

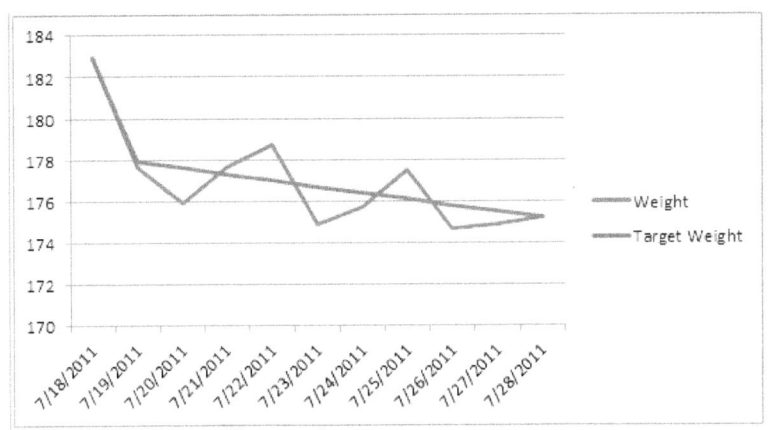

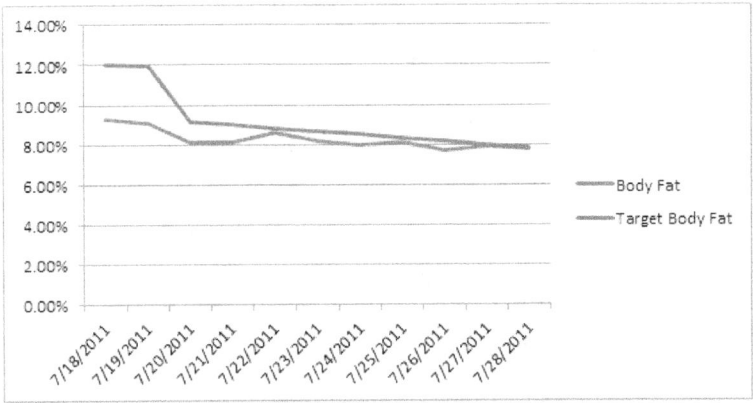

(This spreadsheet, with formulas, is available – just send me a request at bruce@fitforvegas.com and I'll send you information on how to obtain a copy.)

If you're not as geeky as me, just record them somewhere for at least the duration of the program you choose. I've got over four years of data, and I did chart it out. And seriously, it shows me right away how far I've come, especially those days when I need the motivation.

If you liked this idea of using proven measurements to stay on track, let me know by clicking the link or reading the QR code below, and maybe submitting a review. And I'd love to see any comparable measurements methods, like the chart I included here, to see how people track their progress. I know I'm not the only geek that used Excel for pure vanity. Let me know if I'm not alone by posting a review on Amazon, and others can see it and come out of the geek closet too!

http://fitfor.lv/rqPtOA

Science – that extra 10%

Remember the "fat kid pie of cold hard truth"? Remember that little 10% section called "Science"? If you're like most people that are listening to the current fitness trends, that caught your eye right away. The basics are what they are. They don't change much. But there are things that can optimize the impact you have when you're working out. It won't revolutionize your results. But it can make a little difference. I'll give an example to explain why. Think of your car. You're probably roughly aware of the average miles-per-gallon of gas it gets. Let's say your car gets an average of 25 mpg on the highway. Now you might know that having your tires not fully inflated reduces gas mileage because it creates more friction on the road. So does running the air conditioner, as it increases the amount of work on your engine. So does riding with your windows down as it reduces the aerodynamics of the car. So does that mean riding around with full tires, windows up, and the air turned off could make your car get 50 mpg? Heck no; otherwise, you'd see an increase in deodorant sales as gas prices rise. But these things can have an impact of maybe 2 mpg. That's not a lot, but it's something.

The same goes for fitness science. In this section I'll cover three types of fitness "science": exercise science, supplements, and drugs. These can have an incremental impact on your results, but they're not enough to change the results in any massive way. And, unfortunately, these "scientific" approaches often are the areas of fitness that garner the most attention, and thus mislead many fitness seekers from the most important areas of focus and reduce their overall results. I'll cover all of them below, and will even recommend some of them in my programs, but please understand, the fundamentals, like diet and strength training, will be the keys to success. These will just help you save a few "bucks" in gas in your journey to become super-fit by the time you reach Vegas.

Exercise Science

Metabolism. This is the rate at which your body burns calories and uses the nutrients you eat. There are lots of exercises, drugs, and science that "boost" your metabolism. Unfortunately, too many people trying to get fit focus on the techniques to "boost" a metabolism, when in fact, it's the quality of the diet and the workout itself that will most impact fitness. The thing to remember here is the car analogy. You've got a set rate at which your body burns fuel – it's called the basal metabolic rate – and it's largely based on your size. If you weigh more, you burn more. If you weigh less, you burn less. The more work you do, the more calories you burn. The less work you do, the less calories you burn. And no tricky exercise technique is going to change that by more than 20%.

For example, running a mile and walking a mile each burn about the same number of calories for the average person. Why doesn't running burn more? Once again, science helps explain this. Here's a

---

Common Sense Rule #4

Physics apply to fat people too.

$W=Fs$

Work equals the force times the space moved.

physics formula: W=Fs. This is an equation that means "work equals the force times the space moved." The more you weigh the more force is required to move yourself. The further you move, the more work you'll be doing. And that's why running a mile and walking a mile burns very close to the same amount of calories – because you're moving the same weight about the same distance . If you don't believe me, buy a calorie measuring device, like the Body Media FIT, and try it out. Now, to be completely accurate, depending on how fast you run, running will burn a little more because you kind of "push harder" when you run and that causes you to lift your body off the ground just a little bit more than walking. And so while this makes your body work harder, you're still moving your body through the same amount of space, with the same amount of weight, so it roughly equals the same amount of work to run as it does to walk. For example, a 175 pound male will burn about 100 calories walking a mile, and 120 calories running a mile. 20 calories is about how many calories are in a stick of gum. So you can see, the impact is much less significant than one might think. That said, it takes about 15 minutes to walk a mile, and most people can safely run a mile in about 10 minutes.

So you can take advantage of this slight calorie increase and burn a few more calories in a shorter amount of time by doing things like interval training, which speeds up your heart and makes your internal parts of your body "work" harder as the heart pumps faster, the brain sends more electrical signals, and you lungs heave a bit more. Doing things like High Intensity Interval Training (HIIT) takes advantage of these facts. And you'll see I use HIIT in my programs. HIIT moves your body through less space, but increases the work. This means you get in and out of the gym faster. But the reason this is effective is more about simple physics, and less about the more mysterious, and thus often misleading concept, of "boosting" your metabolism.

Supplement Science

I'm going to try and write this up in three paragraphs or less, which is pretty ambitious given how massive the supplement industry is right now. But there are basically only two types of supplements in the fitness industry.

- Those that help you lose weight by "boosting" your metabolism or making you eat less.
- Those that help your body work in the best way possible to meet your goals by giving you good nutrients in an easier-to-get form than in the real world plants or animals that have them.

Most supplements advertised as fat burners or weight loss supplements are in the first camp. And some work a little bit. Caffeine does work. So do supplements like green tea. Some are kind of dangerous, like ephedra. They all have complex reasons for and studies explaining why they work. The thing to remember is they'll at best give you an extra 1 – 5% fat loss due to metabolic increase. This means that an average male, who burns 1500 calories just by being alive, might, at best, add 200 more calories to his daily burn with these supplements. That's something. So in my programs I do suggest some supplements– but I don't bet the farm on them.

The second type of supplement, which includes fish oil, CLA, whey protein, glucosamine, creatine, vitamins, and other minerals, are almost all things you can get by eating the right foods or plants. But the challenge is eating these things at the right time and in the right quantities while trying to do other things like going to work or hanging out with your kids. So these also have a place, because it's easier to scoop out a spoonful of protein than cook a steak right after a workout. So I've included the most proven of these supplements in my programs as well.

Drugs

Mmmm . . . drugs. I know a lot of people who get excited about this topic. Because they think this is where the magic happens. They think if they just had the money to get access to the expensive drugs that they hear of athletes and celebrities using, that they will finally get the fit and toned body they always wanted. The reality is many of these drugs are dangerous, have

> **Common Sense Rule #5**
>
> If buying expensive drugs made you fit, then there would be no fat rich people.

known and unknown negative effects, and as I've said before, can at best impact your fitness by 10%.

These kinds of drugs can seem to have a dramatic effect if you look at professional bodybuilders, but that's only when combined with a long-term strength training commitment and a major focus on diet. So for most of us, just focusing on the 90% of the "fat kid pie" will provide incredible results in a safe, and effective manner. However, the drugs I list below are currently advertised in almost any fitness magazine and website. Despite the mystique about them, they are in fact available to the average citizen. But because of that same mystique, many individuals use them without understanding the consequences, and often, from scam sites that might be selling an even more dangerous substance. I'll share the truth about these drugs with you below. I'll even outline where you can learn more about them. Not so you can use them, but to shine enough practical light on them to explain why they aren't worth the risk. I want to be clear about three things:

1. You don't need them to achieve amazing results.
2. Many of these can have devastating negative effects on your health.
3. At best, they will increase your overall fitness by 10%.

So is it worth it?

These are all grey areas. And the laws keep changing, and I'm no expert in law. So if for you the incremental positive impact is worth all this potential negative risk and the money, then do so at your own risk. You're heading to Vegas, so you should know that you don't always win when you take a gamble.

Anabolic Steroids

Steroids are a broad category for drugs, but in the fitness context, anabolic steroids are drugs that maximize or mimic your body's production of testosterone and its ability to make muscle. It's actually way more complicated than that, but I don't think any of us want to be a biochemist after reading this book.

You can get steroids over-the-counter by ordering "pro hormones" from supplement sites. After you take them, these convert in the body to the same type of steroids you'd have to buy illegally off the street. They are hard on the liver, and they can have pretty major side effects, and each has a program you should follow before, during, and after so you don't end up a total wreck. And for that reason, there's a "cat-and-mouse" game between the manufacturers, who try and find formulas that aren't banned but have the same effect as illegal steroids, and the FDA, which bans these formulas when they have enough proof to show they are unsafe. These over-the-counter oral steroids go by names such as "halodrol," "superdrol,"and "maxlmg." I recommend you go to online forums, like the anabolic forums on sites like anabolicminds.com and do a lot of research and ask a lot of questions so you are at least informed on the safest ways to use them.

Another way to get steroids is from a doctor. There are Hormone Replacement Therapy (HRT) programs, in which an actual MD can diagnose that you have lower than normal testosterone levels. And for most of the docs, "lower than normal" means below the level of a normal 20-year-old. So they'll prescribe a program that pushes your testosterone back into the 20-year-old normal range as a way to help maximize muscle growth and energy. These programs do work. And they aren't that hard to find. But they are quite expensive. Most of them at least require blood tests and have a doctor that will review your results, so they are safer than buying something online and using it with no supervision whatsoever. I'm not going to provide a link to any HRT programs here, but if you search online for hormone replacement therapy you'll likely find a doctor in your area. You can even go to the same site I listed above, anabolicminds.com, and read up on their HRT forums on how to validate doctors. As a guideline, look for the following indicators to know a program is legitimate:

- They charge about 100 – 150 dollars per bottle of testosterone.
- They require blood tests regularly to check the results.
- They also provide other drugs to minimize the negative impacts of the testosterone.

Growth Hormone

This drug has gotten a lot of attention recently, and is one that interests a lot of women as well as men. A few decades ago docs figured out how to manufacture this hormone in a lab, which made getting it way easier than before – which required a human cadaver. Human Growth Hormone (HGH) is almost spoken of as having mystical properties, i.e., it'll help you burn fat faster, gain muscle quicker, it'll make your skin thicker and remove wrinkles. It is a pretty powerful drug. It's also highly regulated, and very expensive. Many of the HRT doctors listed above will prescribe it. Some may also provide effective supplements that aren't HGH, but boost your body's natural production of HGH. If you do this through an HRT doc, they'll at least keep the dosages at a level where it is less likely you'll get the distended bowels and large Cro-Magnon foreheads that high dosages for long periods of time are rumored to cause. As a guideline, look for the following indicators to know an HGH program is legitimate:

- They charge about 300 - 500 dollars for a month's dosage
- It requires a prescription
- It isn't labeled "homeopathic"

HCG – Human Chorionic Gonadotropin

This drug is getting quite a bit of attention in diet circles, as it has an accompanying diet protocol that requires eating about 500 calories a day. A lot of women have tried and had success with this diet. If you've read the earlier parts of the book, you'll realize why that'll definitely work. The diet is squarely in the 70% part of the "fat kid pie of cold hard truth!"

But this drug also helps the body produce testosterone naturally, which is really important if you're already getting it from outside the body through testosterone injections or supplements. It is also known to help the body increase fat loss, but that's most likely due to increasing natural body functions.

If you want HCG, you can get homeopathic versions anywhere. But "homeopathic" is a synonym for "it's kinda what you thought you were buying, but not really." So if you're looking for the regular amount used in prescription programs, then ensure that:

- The dosage is about 250 – 500mg a week
- Costs about 100 – 200 dollars a month.

Again, HRT doctors are known to prescribe this drug as part of their programs.

There's more science to be had. And there are more drugs that help people lose fat and gain muscle. But these are the "big three". The ones most folks hear about most often. And the ones those same people wonder about when they're denying themselves their favorite treat, or busting their ass in the gym.

I hope this answers any lingering doubts about that mystical 10% of the "fat kid pie". And while I'll recommend some aspects of fitness science discussed above in my programs, hopefully you also see that, while this area gets the most attention in fitness magazines, it's actually not the area that requires the most focus in order to get fit.

So, now that you've learned 100% of what's required to get fit, I hope that you are "all-in" for getting fit in time for Vegas, because it is now time to pick a program and get to work.

If you liked this Chapter, please:

Click this link: http://fitfor.lv/w0eD9s

or scan the QR Code below:

The Programs

Below you'll find three programs, each optimally designed for its specific time frame. Each program has three components: the diet, the workout and the science.

- When you've just decided about a week before you leave that you want to look better in your swimsuit, the timeframe I've offered is 7 days.
- When you've given yourself over a month to get ready, the time frame I've offered is 7 weeks.
- When you're thinking way ahead and there are a couple of seasons between you and that next big trip, the time frame I've offered is 7 months.

Choose the program that fits you best, and as long you don't stop too soon, I promise you'll come up a winner.

7 days

Let's face it. You're not going to revolutionize your life in seven days. It took years to get in bad shape and it's at least going to take some months to get in great shape. That said, below is a program that will help you drop 10-15 pounds of water weight, and 2-3 pounds of fat, between today and that next big trip. No matter who you are, walking out to the pool almost 20 pounds lighter will help you enjoy a much better experience. And, since you are coming to Vegas, after all, I've included a few eye-deceiving tricks from the pros to increase your odds of a good time.

7 day Diet

You've got seven days. That means this diet will be aggressive. No cheat days. It'll be designed to drop water weight quick, give you enough energy to work out, and maximize muscle size.

First off – you'll be eating the same thing every day for the next 7 days. The entire diet will be based off that of a contest body-builder getting ready in the last stages of their show, with a reduced carbohydrate footprint to promote water loss.

The serving sizes are based on a 150-200 lb male. If you're a female, or sub-150 lb male, the serving size for you is in [brackets] to the right of the initial item. You'll also notice I include drinking a lot of water in the diet, which might seem counterintuitive to dropping water weight. It's not. By cutting out sodium and carbs, you're helping get the water out of your cells and subcutaneous storage. But you do need to stay hydrated. If your body feels it's getting dehydrated, it'll actually *store* more water which is counter to your goal.

This diet should give you around a 1,200 to 2,000 calorie intake per day depending on body type, which combined with exercise, should net you a 1,000 calorie-a-day deficit. This, if you remember the math from the exercise science chapter, should result in 2 lbs of fat loss by the end of day seven.

The supplements are explained in more detail in the science section.

Breakfast – 6am:

- Coffee with half a pack of sweetener – no cream or milk
- One scoop of whey protein in 16oz of water
- 2 scrambled eggs [1 egg]
- 16 oz of water
- Dandelion root – 1 serving

Mid-morning – 9am:

- At least five fish oil caplets
- 16 oz of water

Lunch

- 6 oz [4 oz] of lean protein (chicken, tuna, or lean game beef)
- 1 cup of broccoli
- 16 oz of water

Mid-day

- 6 oz [4 oz] of lean protein (chicken, tuna, or lean game beef)
- 1 cup of broccoli
- 16 oz of water
- Dandelion root – 1 serving

Pre-workout

- One scoop of whey protein
- 16 oz of water

Post-workout (within the first 20 min after your workout)

- Recovery shake (2:1 carb to protein ration) [half serving]
- 16 oz of water

Dinner

- 6 oz [4 oz] fatty protein (steak, salmon)
- 16 oz of water

Before bed

- One scoop of whey or casein protein
- 16 oz of water

7 day Exercises
With seven days to go, you're going to be working out all but one day between now and show time. Each workout is

designed to increase calorie burn, while retaining muscle mass. I've also added some additional exercises that are explained more in the science section to optimize your short-term impact. Each exercise is linked to an example on the bodybuilding.com website so you can see the proper form. The first number is sets, the last number is repetitions. In other words, 5 X 8 means you do 5 sets of 8 reps. You should choose a weight where you feel like you couldn't do any more reps by the time you finish the last rep of each set. And if you end up doing a couple reps less than what's suggested on your final set, no problem. That means you did it right. Monday – strength training

- Biceps barbell curls: http://fitfor.lv/sKId2V – 5x5
- Triceps press downs: http://fitfor.lv/rZaNMo – 5x8
- Leg extensions: http://fitfor.lv/tEqvBj – 5x8
- Dumbbell flat bench press: http://fitfor.lv/vvDt8X – 5x8
- Lateral raises: http://fitfor.lv/ukCZNs – 5x5
- Straight bar lat pull downs: http://fitfor.lv/sIDgmf – 5x5

Tuesday – cardio

- 20 min HIIT treadmill workout:
    - Minute 1 – easy walk
    - Minute 2 – increase your pace by 2 mph on the treadmill, or to a jogging level where you can easily breathe
    - Minute 3 – increase your pace by an additional 1 mph on the treadmill
    - Minute 4 – increase by 1 mph on the treadmill
    - Minute 5 – decrease your pace to the minute two speed
    - Minute 6 – increase by 1mph on the treadmill
    - Minute 7 – increase by 1mph on the treadmill
    - Minute 8 – increase by 1mph on the treadmill
    - Minute 9 – decrease to the minute two speed
    - Minute 10 – increase by 1mph on the treadmill

- Minute 11 – increase by 1mph on the treadmill
- Minute 12 – increase by 1mph on the treadmill
- Minute 13 – increase by 1mph on the treadmill
- Minute 14 – decrease to the minute two speed
- Minute 15 – increase by 1mph on the treadmill
- Minute 16 – increase by 1mph on the treadmill
- Minute 17 – increase by 1mph on the treadmill
- Minute 18 – increase by 1mph on the treadmill
- Minute 19 – decrease to the minute two speed
- Minute 20++ -- walk and cool down.

Wednesday – strength training

- Same routine as Monday

Thursday – cardio

- Same HIIT routine as Tuesday

Friday – strength training

- Same routine as Monday

Saturday

- Hot Yoga (explained more in the Science section of this program)

Sunday

- Spray Tan

7 day Science

Below are all the supplements listed in the diet section above, and why they are included.

- Fish oil – There are many studies on the benefits of fish oil. The reason I recommend it in my programs is it is an aid in recovery and joint fluidity. You can get this at your supplement store, Costco, or amazon.com – it'll help make sure your joints can handle the days ahead. It can also help fat metabolism.

- Dandelion root – this is a natural diuretic. It'll help drain water from your system quickly, which is why you need to drink a lot of water during this seven day routine to keep critical functions hydrated.
- Whey Protein –this has the essential amino acids that are needed to help your body retain, and possibly build muscle..
- 2:1 carb ratio protein shake – again, go to GNC or search on amazon.com. This ratio gives you the carbs you need to increase your body's insulin to allow the uptake of the nutrients needed to make muscle. There's a short 20-minute window after a workout where you body can best make use of these nutrients for that muscle building.
- HIIT – Most of us don't want to spend more time than needed in the gym. HIIT style training let you get in and get out quickly. Plus, you'll feel less likely to quit a short, but intense, workout than if you were to do a long, slow, jog.
- Hot Yoga – This is a style of yoga that is done in a room at a high temperature. There are many purported benefits of this style of yoga. I recommend it as it will result in losing an extra 2 – 5 pounds of water weight. Find one in your area and follow their safety precautions.
- Spray Tanning – tanning reduces the appearance of body fat due to tricks of light and can highlight what muscle tone you do have. So while I admit this is a pretty cheesy recommendation, it's a legitimate tool to feel great on your vacation. There's a reason body builders and fitness models on stage are tanned. And it's not a sunlamp that gave them that amber look - its spray tan—which is faster, and safer, than a sunlamp. This is entirely optional, but an easy win. To avoid any orange look, find a tanning salon that has a VersaSpa™ brand spray tan, which is fairly well known for a positive, even, 2-minute tan. This is because it uses beet juice and sugar can to result in a bronze color, versus the orange color usually associated with regular spray tans.

By the time you're done with these seven days, you won't be a different person, but you will feel and look a lot better. You'll walk out onto that social stage with more confidence and higher self-esteem than any time before. And who knows, you might even set a foundation that leads to longer workout and diet programs in your future that can have even more dramatic results.

This is almost the perfect lead time to get fit before a trip. With 7 weeks ahead, or 49 days, you can make a pretty amazing transformation.

You will probably be fitter than at least half of the people at the pool during your visit.

How you look will have become an asset to your vacation, not a liability. And for many, including me at one point, that was a major shift.

One result of human evolution is that the body really only does one thing at a time well over a period of a few months: either lose fat or gain muscle. Doing both at the same time can happen, but it takes a lot of time to achieve strong results. The program here is focused on one main goal – dropping off as much fat as possible while gaining modest amounts of muscle.

7 weeks Diet

By signing up for the 7 weeks plan, you've made a big decision. For almost two months you'll be eating from a very limited menu. For 49 days, many times a day, you'll be presented with food that is outside the plan. And, you'll be tempted to tell yourself that one small slip isn't going to affect your overall progress. This is true. The danger is one slip can lead to more, and pretty soon, you're just a few weeks from your trip, and you know you're going to end up looking exactly the same as you did last time you were there.

Success for these 7 weeks isn't determined by this one big decision to commit. It will be determined by making many little decisions each week throughout each day to stick to the plan when you want to deviate.

For these reasons, on the 7-weeks diet, I'm outlining a diet that makes it as easy as possible to avoid making the bad decisions. First - I'm combining a few diets that most people can adhere to. This is because they work well with the full-time work schedules that most of us have. And the "rules" for what you eat are easy to remember and easy to find.

Second – I'm going to ask you to plan your meals. Remember, this is 70% of the "fat kid pie". All day long you are given opportunities to eat something bad for you. All day long you're dealing with stress, work, and life in general. Make eating easy. Take away the guesswork. Cook the main courses for Monday – Friday all at once on Sunday, and put them in Tupperware each day. When you eat out, you'll no longer need to look at menus, because you're going to order "off menu" from one of a few choices. And you'll have your food ready as you go into each day so you'll always know the answer to the "what do I eat next?" question.

Third – this diet is low in simple carbs and sweet substances. Even fruit and low-calorie sweeteners are very low in this plan. This will reduce cravings for carbohydrates and make it easier to stick to the plan. This includes avoiding diet soda. The first three days will be tough, but after that, you'll notice many of the cravings you had in the past will be gone. And it becomes much easier to say "no" to the doughnuts, bagels, and fries that were so tempting before.

Finally, if you've taken the measuring to heart, and I hope you have, then you'll be shooting for a 1,000 calorie a day deficit. This mean you'll want to burn 1,000 calories more than you've eaten. This is the maximum calorie deficit that doesn't eat away too much muscle. Each day, log your food and activities.

If you find you are way under (i.e. you haven't eaten enough) then make the following changes, (in priority order).

- Add an extra scoop of post workout carb/protein drink
- Add an extra scoop of casein protein at night
- Add a handful of almonds at the end of the day

If at some point during the diet, you're falling apart and are convinced you can't make it through the day without some sort of something else than what's on this list, then take the following actions (in priority order).

- Drink a few cups of decaf coffee, each with a small amount of sugar free sweetener
- Drink 16oz of water and take as many fish oil capsules as you want
- Have a one-scoop protein shake
- Have as much broccoli as you want

And try to keep in mind, that in this diet, you'll have two "free periods" on Saturday and Sunday to eat whatever and however much you want. Unlike many diets that provide a "cheat day" or a "cheat meal" spreading these meals over two days provides extra carbs for muscle building, as well as more opportunity to enjoy the foods you've been craving. And by limiting the timeframe to two hours, you'll be surprised how much you can eat, and how satisfying it is. I typically have time left over, and will have put down several burgers, pizza, and close to a dozen doughnuts on my "free meals". Done right, you'll be looking forward to eating clean again starting on Monday.

Weeks 1 – 4
Monday – Friday you'll eat the same meal(s) each day.

Breakfast – 6am:

- Coffee with half a pack of sweetener – no cream or milk
- 16 oz of water

Mid-morning – 9am:

- At least five fish oil caplets
- 16 oz of water

Note: If you have trouble making it to the through the day to the first meal, take more fish oil tablets and drink more water one or two more times in the morning. The combination can prove satiating, and get you through any hunger pains.

Lunch

- 6 oz [4 oz] of lean protein (chicken, tuna, or lean game beef)
- 1 cup of broccoli
- 16 oz of water

Mid-day

- 6 oz [4 oz] of lean protein (chicken, tuna, or lean game beef)
- 1 cup of broccoli
- 16 oz of water

Pre-workout

- One scoop of whey protein
- 16 oz of water

Post-workout (within the first 20 min after your workout)

- Recovery shake (2:1 carb to protein ration) [half serving]
- 16 oz of water

Dinner

- 12 oz [4 oz] of fatty protein (steak, salmon)

- 16 oz of water

Before bed

- Two scoops of whey or casein protein
- One handful of almonds
- At least five fish oil capsules
- 16 oz of water

Saturday and Sunday

Breakfast – 6am:

- Coffee with half a pack of sweetener – no cream or milk
- 3 eggs and 2 sausage links [1 egg and 1 link]
- 16 oz of water

Mid-morning – 9am:

- At least five fish oil caplets
- 16 oz of water

Lunch

- 6 oz [4 oz] of lean protein (chicken, tuna, or lean game beef)
- 1 cup of broccoli
- 16 oz of water

Mid-day

- 6 oz [4 oz] of lean protein (chicken, tuna, or lean game beef)
- 1 cup of broccoli
- 16 oz of water

Pre-workout

- One scoop of whey protein
- 16 oz of water

Post-workout (within the first 20 min after your workout)

- Recovery shake (2:1 carb to protein ration) [half serving]
- 16 oz of water

Dinner

- Free meal – eat whatever you want but:
- Only give yourself 2 hours to eat so you limit the damage
- Have at least 6 oz [4 oz] of protein in this meal

Weeks 5 – 7
Breakfast – 6am:

- Coffee with half a pack of sweetener – no cream or milk
- 16 oz of water

Mid-morning – 9am:

- At least five fish oil caplets
- 16 oz of water
- Dandelion root – 1 serving

Lunch

- 6 oz [4 oz] of lean protein (chicken, tuna, or lean game beef)
- 1 cup of broccoli
- 16 oz of water

Mid-day

- 6 oz [4 oz] of lean protein (chicken, tuna, or lean game beef)
- 1 cup of broccoli
- 16 oz of water
- Dandelion root – 1 serving

Pre-workout

- One scoop of whey protein
- 16 oz of water

Post-workout (within the first 20 min after your workout)

- Recovery shake (2:1 carb to protein ration) [half serving]
- 16 oz of water

Dinner

- 12 oz [4 oz] of fatty protein (steak, salmon)
- 16 oz of water

Before bed

- Two scoops of whey or casein protein
- At least five fish oil capsules
- 16 oz of water

Saturday and Sunday

Breakfast – 6am:

- Coffee with half a pack of sweetener – no cream or milk
- 3 eggs and 2 sausage links [1 egg and 1 link]
- 16 oz of water

Mid-morning – 9am:

- At least five fish oil caplets
- 16 oz of water

Lunch

- 6 oz [4 oz] of lean protein (chicken, tuna, or lean game beef)
- 1 cup of broccoli
- 16 oz of water

Mid-day

- 6 oz [4 oz] of lean protein (chicken, tuna, or lean game beef)
- 1 cup of broccoli
- 16 oz of water

Pre-workout

- One scoop of whey protein
- 16 oz of water

Post-workout (within the first 20 min of your workout)

- Recovery shake (2:1 carb to protein ration) [half serving]
- 16 oz of water

Dinner

- 12 oz [4 oz] of lean protein (chicken, tuna, or lean game beef)
- 1 cup of broccoli
- 16 oz of water

7 week Exercises

The exercises below are designed to increase fat loss, but focuses on muscle groupings with a split that helps growth. It does this by giving just enough time for each muscle group to recover and rebuild before you hit it again. More on the rationale behind these choices is explained in the 7-week science section.

These exercises will work to tone the right parts for both women and men, as these are "fundamental" exercises that work major muscle groups. And each is linked to bodybuilding.com to show the proper form. As in the 7-day program, the first number is the number of sets, and the second number is the number of reps performed each set. Use as much weight as you can to just finish the number of reps.

For weeks 1-4 you'll do the first number of reps. For weeks 5-7 you'll do the second number of reps in [brackets].

Monday – Chest

- Incline Dumbbell Press: http://fitfor.lv/t6zKo7 - 4x8[15]
- Dumbbell Flies: http://fitfor.lv/rvqCCM - 4x8[15]
- Dumbbell Bench Press: http://fitfor.lv/vvDt8X - 3x8[12]
- Cable Crossovers: http://fitfor.lv/vItLEL - 7x8[12]

Tuesday – Arms and Abs

- 20 crunches: http://fitfor.lv/tRGs1B - 3x10 [15]
- 20 reverse crunches: http://fitfor.lv/u5vUfj – 3x10 [15]
- Close-Grip Bench Press: http://fitfor.lv/t6lJAf - 4x8 [12]
- Dips: http://fitfor.lv/tBgna2 - 3x8[12]
- Lying Triceps Press: http://fitfor.lv/rZaNMo - 7 x8 [12]
- Barbell curls: http://fitfor.lv/sKId2V - 4x8 [12]
- Hammer curls: http://fitfor.lv/rxCf74 - 3x8 [12]
- Preacher curls: http://fitfor.lv/rCKEMx - 7x 8 [12]

Wednesday

- Rest or Cardio (Optional)

Thursday – Back and Shoulders

- Lat Pull downs: http://fitfor.lv/sIDgmf - 3x8[12]
- Bent Over Barbell Rows: http://fitfor.lv/toSUML - 3x8[12]
- Seated Cable Rows: http://fitfor.lv/tBVr9a - 3x8[12]
- Barbell Pullovers: http://fitfor.lv/sbCWMz - 7x8[12]

- Upright rows: http://fitfor.lv/suiOo1 - 4x8[12]
- Front Dumbbell Raises: http://fitfor.lv/v5clzg - 3x8[12]
- Side Lateral Raises: http://fitfor.lv/ukCZNs - 3x8[12]

Friday – Legs and Abs

- 20 crunches: http://fitfor.lv/tRGs1B -3x10 [15]
- 20 reverse crunches: http://fitfor.lv/u5vUfj – 3x10 [15]
- Lying Leg Curls: http://fitfor.lv/tW8Vnl - 4x10[15]
- Deadlift: http://fitfor.lv/v2ksTm - 4x10[15]
- Standing Calf Raises: http://fitfor.lv/taGKnw - 4x10[12]
- Measure – weight, body fat, body circumference.

Saturday

- Cardio – (optional)

Sunday

- Rest.

7 week Science

For the diet, there are a few things going on. You'll notice the absence of breakfast during the week. This is borrowed from an idea of fasting for weight loss, documented in a fitness book called "Eat-Stop-Eat" by Brad Pilon. It recommends a style of eating called "intermittent fasting" and if you want more logic behind the approach than I am about to give you, read that e-book. However, a fitness enthusiast named Martin Berkhan has modified this diet to focus on lean muscle gains. His website leangains.com is a great resource for even more information on why this diet works. However, the bottom line is that this approach makes it easy for the average human to keep a calorie deficit, as it times eating around the blocks of the day where you're most likely to cheat—the evenings. I've modified both Brad and Martin's diets for one that delivers excellent results, but is even more conducive to the every-day busy individual. Also, the food choices follow the "Paleo Diet" very closely in that they are mostly slow-digesting carbs like veggies, with the fast-digesting carbs only right after your workout. I've also included several supplements to add that extra 10% each with various supplements:

- Fish oil – get this at your supplement store, Costco, or amazon.com – it'll help make sure your joints can handle the days ahead.
- Dandelion root – this is a natural diuretic. It'll help drain water from your system quickly, which is why you need. To drink a lot of water during this seven-week routine to keep critical functions hydrated. In this program it's introduced during the last three weeks.
- Whey protein – this has the essential amino acids that are needed to tell your body it needs to hold onto muscle.
- 2:1 Carb ratio protein shake –go to GNC or search on amazon.com. This ratio gives you the carbs you need to increase the body's insulin to allow the uptake of the nutrients needed to make muscle. There's a short 20-minute window after a workout where your body can best make use of these nutrients for that muscle retention.

The exercises are inspired by a style of training called Fascia-Stretch Training 7, or FST-7. The "7" refers to the 7 set exercises that show up in some of the work outs. The idea behind this program is that it really builds a "pump" of blood into the muscles that makes them swollen and engorged. This makes your workout feel awesome while also helping give the muscles room to grow. This program is used by many of the leading fitness professionals, and its creator, Hany Rambod, trains many of the best.

Also – cardio is optional. If you do it, the reason you're doing it is for cardiovascular health, or heart health. Or just because you enjoy running, swimming, cycling, etc. With the diet you're following, and the workout routine, you won't need additional cardio to meet your goals.

7 months

Congratulations! By choosing the 7-month program, you've got a chance to fundamentally change the way you look. A major transformation is possible. You can be one of the top ten fittest people anywhere you go. You can be one of the first people in your circle of friends to break through the "I just workout" barrier into the realm of the super-fit, ripped and toned. It'll show in your appearance at work, at home, and of course, on vacation. Get the camera ready. These are the Facebook pics you've been waiting for.

But first – this is a long haul, not a sprint. Most people don't make it. If they did, you'd know more fit people, right? How will this experience be different? Well, first, you know more about why this stuff will work because you've read and educated yourself. Second – you're going to measure your progress which will put right in your face how far forward you've come and have far back you may have slipped. And third – I offer these two tips for you to keep in mind to help you stay on track for 7 months:

- Try and be perfect. You goal is perfection. Do every diet to the letter, every workout as prescribed. Don't skip, don't cheat. If you want to change something, change it on Sunday and make it part of the plan. But stick to the plan.

- You won't be exactly perfect. Life will happen. Remember what I said in the chapter on the "the basics": You have to do these things more days than you don't. If you're doing that, you will achieve the phenomenal results. So, if you misstep, go back to trying to be perfect, and you'll quickly average out to awesome.

7 month Diet

No matter who you are, you can't follow a super strict diet for 7 months. So this diet needs to be based on a solid foundation of principles. The first is periodization, or focusing on one thing at a time for a long enough period of time. That means this diet will be broken into four 7-week parts.

- For the first 7 weeks we're going to focus on fat loss, or cutting. This will get you lean and ready to build additional muscle.
- The second 7 weeks will focus on building as much muscle as possible in a short time.
- The third 7 weeks will focus on making that muscle "mature" to keep the muscle you just gained.
- And finally, for the last 7 weeks we'll do an aggressive cut to get you lean for your vacation.

Again, this diet and the supplements are explained more in the science section. And the same format applies as the other programs. It's designed for an average male. But if you're under 150 lbs, or a female, the portions are in [brackets] next to each entry.

First 7 weeks
- Follow the same diet as the 7-week diet plan. It's already tailor-made for cutting.

Second 7 weeks

Monday – Friday you'll eat the same meal(s) each day.

Breakfast – 6 am:

- Coffee with half a pack of sweetener – no cream or milk
- 16 oz of water

Mid-morning – 9 am:

- At least five fish oil caplets
- 16 oz of water

Lunch

- 12 oz [6 oz] of lean protein (chicken, tuna, or lean game beef)
- 1 cup of broccoli
- 16 oz of water

Mid-day

- 12 oz [6 oz] of lean protein (chicken, tuna, or lean game beef)
- 1 cup of broccoli
- 16 oz of water

Pre-workout

- Two scoops of whey protein
- 16 oz of water

Post-workout (within the first 20 min of your workout)

- Recovery shake (2:1 carb to protein ration) [half serving]
- 16 oz of water

Dinner

- 18 oz [6 oz] of fatty protein (steak, salmon)

- 16 oz of water

Before bed

- Two scoops of whey or casein protein
- One handful of almonds
- Two tablespoons of peanut butter
- At least five fish-oil capsules
- 16 oz of water

Saturday and Sunday

Breakfast – 6 am:

- Coffee with half a pack of sweetener – no cream or milk
- 3 eggs and 2 sausage links [1 egg and 1 link]
- 2 cups [1 cup] of steel cut oatmeal
- 16 oz of water

Midmorning – 9am:

- At least five fish oil caplets
- 16 oz of water

Lunch

- 6 oz [4 oz] of lean protein (chicken, tuna, or lean game beef)
- 1 cup of broccoli
- 1 cup [1/2 cup] of brown rice
- 16 oz of water

Mid-Day

- 6 oz [4 oz] of lean protein (chicken, tuna, or lean game beef)
- 1 cup of broccoli
- 16 oz of water

Pre-workout

- Two scoops of whey protein
- 16 oz of water

Post-workout (within the first 20 min after your workout)

- Recovery shake (2:1 carb to protein ration) [half serving]
- 16 oz of water

Dinner

- Free meal – eat whatever you want but:
- Only give yourself 2 hours to eat so you limit the damage
- Have at least 12 oz [6 oz] of protein in this meal

Third 7 weeks
- This is the "reprieve" period, where you take a bit of a break, but won't backtrack
- You will follow a diet that has a few simple rules
- Eat at least 5 meals a day.
- Don't start eating until 1 pm.
- Stop eating by 9 pm.
- Each meal should have at least 6 oz [4 oz] of protein (eggs, chicken, fish, beef, etc) and 1 cup of vegetables
- Don't eat any starchy grains or dairy – no cheese, no rice, no bread
- Schedule two hours on Saturday and Sunday to cheat with whatever you want. Even a fat cold pizza.

Fourth 7 weeks
- Follow the same diet as the 7-week diet plan – it is already tailor-made for cutting.

7 month Exercises
7 months. That's a long time to do anything you read in a book. I don't care if that book is the best fitness book ever written, a self-help manual written by the Dalai Lama himself, or even the Bible. It's a long period of time to just be managed by an inanimate object.

So this is one area where I'd recommend getting creative.

First – you can start with the workouts recommended in the 7-week plan. That's perfectly acceptable. This is a solid foundation, and will help you through your first 7-week cut.

But after 7 weeks, you will start to get bored. You'll start to slack. Your workouts will be run-of-the-mill and you won't make the progress you think you should.

However, if you're willing to make the investment for the 7 month exercise plan, I strongly recommend what I mentioned in the introductory chapter on exercising in general: Get a personal trainer. Or try CrossFit™. Make sure your trainer is fit themselves, and meet once a week. Ask him (or her) to give you copies of the workout. Use those workouts when you're not training with him. You'll only do this for the first 7 weeks. After the first 7 weeks, you'll have one or two workouts for each major body part. This approach has worked for countless people.

7 month Science
There are three major scientific principles in use in this plan.

- The body is made to do one thing at a time really well. For this reason, we've got a typical cut/bulk/maintain/cut cycle for this 7-month program. I say "typical" because if you see a really fit person, ask them if they are currently cutting, bulking or maintaining. They'll have an answer.
- The diet is using principles from the same two diets mentioned in the 7-week program: intermittent fasting and the "Paleo Diet". Both have been optimized for muscle gain and cut depending on the focus of the 7-week period.
- The workout routine is the same as the 7-week plan. That said, one additional rule to follow during the 7-week muscle gain period is to lift the heaviest weight you can,

and increase the amount of time you rest. This puts a severe load on the muscles, and pushes the FST-7™ routine created by Hany Rambod to focus even more on increased muscle size.

The supplements suggested in the 7-week program are also used here.

One of these three programs I've outlined should reasonably fit the time frame between now and your next vacation, plus or minus a day, week, or a month or two. If the diets, workouts, and science seem helpful, let me know by clicking the link below.

http://fitfor.lv/umCvBy

The self-feeding fitness machine – the fitness industry explained.

With the programs above, covered in just a few short pages, I'm promising amazing results. This may seem to defy common sense. If it were that simple, why are there so many articles on fitness in magazines, TV ads, TV shows, diet programs, trying to get our attention every day? If it's as easy as what I just said, wouldn't everybody be doing it and wouldn't the fitness industry come to a grinding halt?

Well, no, it won't. Not because I missed important facts. But because of one simple truth: the industry is set up to keep itself alive. It's not some evil plot. I love the fitness industry. I've been a consumer, contributor, and participant for decades. Rather, it's just a natural business process. Here's why:

- Supplement manufacturers keep doing research into new methods to have a positive impact, even if it's just marginal, because if they do they'll sell more products.
- Magazines and other media need good sales figures to attract advertising revenue, so they keep writing articles about awesome new breakthroughs that are new and novel to get your interest.
- Gyms keep changing their programs and adopting new classes and machines to keep people interested and paying their monthly dues.
- Fitness pros and bloggers need content to keep you coming to their site to sell product and increase page rankings on the internet, so they're always looking for a new development to talk about.

But day-to-day, and year-over-year, 90% of the "fat kid pie of cold hard truth" basically stays the same. These basics haven't changed that much in the last 50 years. But the points above form a vicious circle where each step feeds into the other. The end result is that an incredibly massive amount of information and products are produced almost daily to help people be fit. And that's just from the products that are actually positive in their impact and aren't 99% hype. So there's really no hope that anyone with a real life can wade through it all to the barebones, most effective, and simplest approach.

That's what I've tried to do here. I don't want to keep you coming back. I just want to find the most effective way to communicate about the most important facts to help people reach their fitness goals, so they can get on with their lives. And get on with fun stuff. Like a great Vegas vacation.

If you liked this Chapter, please:

Click this link: http://fitfor.lv/rteVOx

or scan the QR Code below:

Why Vegas?

If you've made it this far, you've probably realized that there's nothing specifically unique to Vegas in these approaches. I've chosen this title because it is the single most sought after vacation destination for the largest demographic world-wide. It also has a "day life" scene that has exploded over the last few years. Night clubs are still raging on, but there are now "day clubs," pool versions of night clubs, that are taking over the scene. And what a great idea that was. It's all the fun of a night club, but you can get a tan and see people wearing less clothing. I don't think this scene will end anytime soon.

The second reason I've chosen Vegas is because as a major vacation destination, it's also one where a lot of people reflect back on their current lifestyles as they return. The vast majority of self-promises to get fit either happen immediately following a vacation or right before planning the next one. While I'd love more people to get fit to just have a better daily life, having a rewarding target, like an awesome vacation, is a key motivator.

It was for me. Many years ago I was sitting by the pool one day, balancing a plate of burger and fries on my belly and trying to find a sweet potato french fry I dropped down my lap. It was stuck in a fat fold of my belly. That wasn't the last time I ate a burger or a sweet potato fry. But it was the last time my fat folds served as crumb catchers on a vacation. I know that's not the most emotionally heart-wrenching tale of overcoming human tragedy, but it did suck. And I know I'm not alone. The stuff in this book worked for me, and many others, and I'm sure it'll work for you.

If you liked this Chapter, please:

Click this link: http://fitfor.lv/rFSkMT

or scan the QR Code below:

The real about me page

Who am I? Well, I'll let you in on a secret: my name isn't really Bruce Agate. The reason I've written under this pseudonym isn't because I don't believe in and am not proud of the content. I am. But I don't want my whole world to be about fitness. I have a real job. A real life. A real family. Fitness pros are awesome, dedicated people. But most, whether intentionally or not, become their own brand. I wanted to find a way to share decades of research, feedback from family and friends, and experience of fitness pros, with a broader audience-- without becoming a fitness pro myself.

That said, I've invested more time into this industry than most fitness pros I know. I've been a consumer since I was in my early teens back in the 80s. I've trained family, friends, and clients. I've developed my own supplement stacks, diets, and tested them with these same people. I've contributed heavily to online forums. I've helped people train for fitness contests. I've followed fitness contest regimes myself. I've probably read, tested, and commented on over 1,000 fitness e-books, print books, and blogs over these years, and read every major fitness magazine and online site in that time. And man, did I ever waste a lot of time, money, hopes, and dreams on stuff that really didn't work in the long run.

Through all that, I've found a plan that keeps me between 4% and 8% body fat (by hydrostatic testing) year-round. I eat wonderfully tasting, but horribly fattening foods in disgusting amounts every once in a while. I can bench 300 pounds. I can run ten miles without concern. And when I walk around in my workout gear, I routinely get asked for fitness advice by total strangers. And yet, I work a full-time professional career that has received attention in major media as one of the top ten most stressful jobs in the industry. I have a girlfriend that I love spending time with. And I have family and friends who are way more important to me than my fitness routine.

So am I qualified to write a book like this? You let me know. Click a link on each chapter to quickly tell me what you think. Write a review and email me at bruce@fitforvegas.com. Let me know if this book has helped. I promise if you take the time to do that, I'll take the time to listen, give you a personal reply, and a gift as well.

If you liked this Chapter, please:

Click this link: http://fitfor.lv/rFSkMT

or scan the QR Code below:

Get Fit for Vegas

By Bruce Agate

bruce@fitforvegas.com

Copyright 2011 © Bruce Agate

www.ingramcontent.com/pod-product-compliance
Lightning Source LLC
Chambersburg PA
CBHW060205290526
45789CB00003B/1171